It Ain't No Darn Diet Book

It Ain't No Darn Diet Book

Melissa Mathis

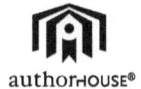

authorHOUSE®

AuthorHouse™
1663 Liberty Drive
Bloomington, IN 47403
www.authorhouse.com
Phone: 1-800-839-8640

First published by AuthorHouse   11/19/2011

ISBN: 978-1-4670-9450-4 (sc)
ISBN: 978-1-4670-9425-2 (ebk)

Library of Congress Control Number: 2011919620

Printed in the United States of America

MY CREDENTIALS:

At Seventeen-years-old, I got the best advice from my naturally thin friend. "Melissa, you know, you should just diet and exercise and then you would lose weight."

"Oh. My. Gosh! Really? I had never thought of that! You have just inspired me to transform my life, oh ye of size three jeans. Bless you!"

I'm not a doctor and I don't have any letters after my name. I am thirty-one-years-old and have been on diets for the last twenty-two years. Yep, if you did the math right, I started at nine. You name the diet or pill, and, more than likely, I have done it. I have done the shakes, the soups, the pills, the calculations . . . and, they worked . . . And then they didn't. Finally, I found the "secret". It ain't no darn secret, just like it ain't no darn diet. It's a whole lot of little things that will literally change your life. Without yo-yo dieting, pill-popping, lap band, gastric bypass (or any other bypass), I have lost from over THREE-HUNDRED pounds to one-hundred-and-seventy-five pounds, and counting! I stopped listening to well-meaning-never-been-fat people, and started listening to myself.

At times I may sound harsh, but now is the time to set aside your excuses and succeed. I know, I know. Genetics, depression, sickness, divorce, money's tight. This is why you packed on the pounds. Whatever the reason, you got yourself here, now let's get you out.

*MAKE PLANS FOR THE FUTURE . . . START NOW

I always thought, "If I can lose a hundred pounds, I can do anything". Then, one day, I had lost that hundred pounds. And I was lost.

I stopped losing, *majorly*, plateau-ing for a LONG time. I had set my major goal for losing a hundred pounds because, at over three-hundred, that seemed to be the biggest I could dream, something impossible. So, because that was the only dream I made, I was lost after I got there. I had a lot more to go, but my goal had been set for a hundred. I had to start over by creating new goals. My biggest problem was that I believed my whole world, my whole life, would amazingly change and become perfect when I lost the weight. But . . . it didn't.

Besides me, my family and friends, the rest of the world didn't know of my *huge* accomplishment. It wasn't as if I could go around with a shirt that said, **'I may be big now, but you should have seen me before!'** The worst was when a new person started at my gym and offered *me* advice because she had lost ten pounds. She thought that I had gained **up** to what I had actually lost **down** to. That killed me. I had to be stronger, and push myself all the harder, and most of all, I had to realize that **my weight wasn't the *problem* of my life, it was a symptom.**

I had to stop, look inside myself, and figure out what had led me to gain all that weight in the first place. It is rarely just one thing, so if you figure out one, keep on digging. I can honestly tell you, this was harder than losing my first hundred pounds.

It requires a *ton* of introspection, realizations and acceptance of my part, my responsibility and my BLAME in how my life had turned out. Yeah, there were things that I went through that I didn't expect. You don't enter a situation expecting everything to blow up in your face. However, I made the choice to enter into that situation. Regardless of the outcome, it was my choice to be there in the first place. The situation wasn't the issue. I could spend the rest of my life feeling like a victim but, why was I there in the first place? Could it have been my screwed up self-esteem? Just as I chose to be in the situation, I also had the choice to be the victim or the conqueror. I had played the role of victim long enough. I made the conscious decision to become the conqueror. In making that choice that meant that I had to let go of all the excuses I made for myself in my role as the victim. I no longer had a passive role in my failure or success.

You may go through things or have gone through things that are out of your control, but you *are* in control of how you *respond* to the situation. Problem was, I had lost my built-in excuse for failure; I lost my built-in excuse as the victim. I had lost the excuse that it wasn't my fault that I wasn't a success; the world was against me because I was fat. In my mind, my failures were not my fault, but it was the fault of society for not accepting that a fat person could be successful. That was not a fun day, but, it was a total AHA moment. It didn't end there. Once you realize the problems, the reasons, you have to begin the process of remedying it.

My first Aha moment, the moment that it just 'clicked' that something had to change was in my car on the freeway. I had been out with a few friends. I had learned to use humor as a defense mechanism. You know, crack the joke on yourself before others can. It takes the fun out of putting someone down if they think it doesn't hurt you. To an outsider, it would seem that it had been a great night. I was surrounded by a group of people, making them laugh with my fat jokes. Everybody was smiling and laughing.

It is amazing that I can remember instances from before that you would think would lead me to the Aha moment but they didn't. No one had made fun of me that night, but me. Nobody gave me the 'I'm in a zoo' look. For all intents and purposes, it was a good night.

I was driving my car home. It had rained just enough to make the roads slippery. A car pulled over on me and when I swerved to miss it, my car hydroplaned.

I just barely missed going over the edge of the ramp, into a deep drop. I could have crashed and died, but I didn't.

I sat in the emergency only lane, my hands shaking, my heart pounding, crying; not because I was almost in an accident that could have killed me, but because I *wasn't* in an accident that killed me. My moment, my choice, was then. I felt I had to choose; either I lose weight and take control of my life or take my life.

Come to your AHA moment *now* and take control of your life, of your success. Go forth with the knowledge that your success is in your hands.

Be an active participant in your life!

*Make a list of how it feels/ what I have kept/keep myself from because of my weight

There is a section in your journal to record this. Include everything you can think of, even if it is from years ago.

The following are some of the things that I included in my journal:

WHAT SUCKED/WHAT I HAVE KEPT MYSELF FROM BECAUSE OF MY WEIGHT:

- See-Saw on the playground . . . need I say more?
- As a kid, being fat doesn't hurt just you, but your family as well. There were times that my family would cry with me because I had been made fun of in school. As pathetic as it may seem, I found a journal I had written in seventh grade that said, "Today was a good day. I only got made fun of once." I read that journal nearly fifteen years later and cried.

- Track. I was GREAT at hurdles. When my P.E. coach told me that I should try out for the track team, well, being fat all my life, it was like a dream. Then the nightmares flooded my mind. Visions of people watching me, the fat chick, running down the track. The whispers that would go through the crowd. The knowing looks on my competitors when they looked at me, knowing that they had zero chance of losing to me. So, I never tried.

- Speech. I love to talk. It's one thing I know I'm good at. I wanted to join the speech team or drama so badly, but, why would anybody want to listen to me, the fat kid? As far as drama was concerned, I would be darned before I let myself be put into all the "fat girl" roles; no 'Mrs Claus' thank you very much! All I needed was to display my fat for all the school to watch!

- Kid's clothes: It would have been great if, when I was a kid, I could wear *kid's* clothes. When I was growing up, it seemed as if the clothing industry had no idea that there were big kids out there that needed to wear *kids'* clothes. As a result, I had to wear adult size clothes. Instead of looking like I was getting dressed for a day of school, in fifth grade I looked like I was getting dressed for a day at the office.

- Swimming parties: When you are a teen and your thigh is the size of most of your friends' torsos, parading around in a bathing suit is so not anybody's idea of fun!

- Desks with attached chairs: Who in the world created these torture devices and thought, "Hey, middle school is, socially, the hardest time in a tween/teen's life. Let's put these in their classes!"??? I would look around and see girls in my class who were actually able to sit AND put their legs up so their knees were to their chest between the chair and the table, while I was sucking in and still having the roll of fat being cut in half by the edge of the table. But, these *nice, oh so nice,* creators of this "desk" thought to be kind to the larger kids and put at least one of the "bigger kid's desk" in each classroom. Same creation, larger proportions. Two problems. First, if there was more than just one "bigger" kid, you are competing with them to get that desk. Two, the skinny kids didn't realize the reason for that bigger desk and thought it was better to sit there. Yeah, like I am going to walk my 12-year-old heft up to them and say, "Hey, I like breathing and that desk actually allows it. Can we trade?" Oh, Hell-o NO!

- Health Education: This is a class that is required to graduate, and, as much as I understand the reasoning of it, information on how to take care of yourself, proper hygiene and all, the part that totally stunk was when they would talk about healthy eating and . . . here it comes . . . OBESITY!

All the kids in class would turn and look at me. I could not suck in my stomach enough!

- Job interviews: Forget about wearing something that makes you feel confident, you're more concerned with just trying to find something that fits. It's so not impressive when you walk into an interview wearing a sky-blue moo-moo.

- Dancing: I LOVE TO DANCE! I love, love, love it! You feel the beat of the music and it just calls for you to shake your groove thing! But when your "milkshake" is more like a gelato shop, and you're "belly-dancing" keeps going when the music stops, it's not so fun. And looking at the "girls" around you wearing the same amount of material all over them that you have on your left thigh . . . again, not so fun.

- Group pictures: These suck. Period. When it seems that everyone around you is half your size. Have you ever noticed how *somehow,* you are always in the back? Coincidence? I think NOT!

- Clothes shopping (especially with "normal-sized" friends): It sucks that one of the few things that fits is the fitting room. It sucks to have to shop below the "Plus Size" neon pink sign that pretty much states, "fat woman shopping below!" to the rest of the store. And, the idea of actually saying our clothing size to *anybody* is out of the question, as if telling them our clothing size is going to magically make them suddenly realize how big we are. Really? As if they can't already tell. There is no choice of what you want, it is what fits, or at least stretches to the "right" size.

- Airplane seatbelts: I dreaded the moment we had to put that belt on. Well, it wasn't so much the seat belt as much as the extender that I had to ask for. How humiliating it was to have to ask the flight attendant for the extender and her not hearing so I had to ask again, louder, for all the people around to hear. Yea! Fun . . . good fun . . .
- Boots: I LOVE knee high boots. I think they look so sexy . . . just not on me! The ones that had a zipper that would not zip up all the way, or the ones with stretch would go from knee highs to anklets throughout the day, and if they didn't have a zipper or stretch, they weren't fitting over my calves.
- Pretty panties: Lacey, hi-cut, silk, G-strings . . . never met 'em. Granny-panties were my best friend.
- Eating lunch alone in the library because I was too shy, too ashamed to ask other kids if I could eat lunch with them.

One time I will never forget was when I was in seventh grade. It was the Sadie Hawkins dance and I had already assumed that I wasn't going to go. Why would I dare ask a boy to go to the dance with me? Why would I even risk the chance of being made fun of, risk the surety of the humiliation of rejection. Oh yeah . . . and a girl named Kelly(names have been changed to protect the innocent/guilty). She was the popular girl. The one that every boy wanted to date and every girl (including me) wanted to be.

Kelly wore the most stylish clothes, was smart, but not *too* smart, perfect hair, perfect nails, and ran around with a group of just-next-to-perfect girls. I didn't even begin to fool myself into thinking that I could ever be good enough to fit into her group, but you can't keep a girl from dreaming.

Four days before the dance, she and two of her friends approached me in the library. Kelly came and sat next to me at the table and, as her friends joined, told me, "Melissa, you know Jason don't you?" Jason was in the boy version of Kelly's group. Popularity came naturally to them. I had the *hugest* crush on Jason. At the time, I was just shocked that *she* was sitting at my table. I didn't pay attention to the looks between her and her friends. I just nodded. "Jason wants you to ask him to the dance. He told me, right Cindy?" As always, Cindy agreed with her. Stupid me. Even though it made *zero* sense, I believed her.

I met him where she told me to meet him. After I asked him, right before he could answer, all her, and *his* friends came out from around the corner laughing. Jason never said yes or no. The most pathetic thing was that they weren't doing it to be mean to *me*, they were playing a joke on *him*. Jason didn't know anything about it. The joke wasn't on me;

_I_ was the joke. After that, a _joke_ is all I thought I would ever be.

These are just some samples. Think hard. Write down things you have kept yourself from in the past and things you keep yourself from now. No matter how long ago it happened, if you remember it, it had an effect on you. WRITE IT!

*Make a list of reasons to stay fat

Yes, I am serious. There ARE reasons to stay fat. How awesome is it that there are such lowered expectations for large people. I mean, isn't it like _way_ easier to not attempt something difficult because, "Hey, I'm fat. They'll never take me serious." You never risk a 'fail' because you never have to take the chance. Congratulations! You have your very own, handy-dandy, built-in excuse. This is a reality check, a be-honest-with-yourself, no-holds-barred, get-real, look-deep moment. Accept your blame and your responsibility for your place in life. This is _the_ most important key to your success. _I_ can't _make_ you lose weight. _Nobody_ can but YOU! Record these reasons in the section for it in your journal.

This is actually one of the harder parts for you to figure out. I mean, we _know_ if we had the choice of having someone grant our wishes, being thin would _definitely_ rank right up there at the top, but, amazingly, there are reasons to stay fat.

Melissa Mathis

Here are some of the reasons from my journal and some of my friends' journals.

Reasons to stay fat:

* * I surprise people when I actually do something that requires intelligence
* * People expect way less of me so I don't have to work as hard
* * (From a friend in a troubled marriage) I won't have other guys check me out so I won't have the temptation to cheat
* * I can't afford the healthy food (*amazingly,* healthy food does seem more expensive!)
* * With all the stress in my life, if I try dieting, I will go insane!
* * I've tried dieting before and failed. All I need is to fail again and feel even *more* like a loser.

*The second greatest part of this experience is the first two days. You MUST eat how you normally eat. If you normally eat a Big Mac for lunch, eat a Big Mac. If you eat two king-size candy bars a day, EAT two king-size candy bars. But, yep, there is a big, cellulite filled butt in there, BUT you *have* to track your calories. Also, if you eat something that is not prepackaged, like cereal, you need to pour the normal amount you eat into a bowl and then put that into a measuring cup and figure out the calories. An average serving size, according to the box, is 2/3 a cup.

Don't lie to yourself. YOU DO NOT BENEFIT ANY BY LYING TO YOURSELF! 'Cause, really, lying to yourself has been so successful in the past. "Man! The dryer really shrank my jeans!" Let's be real and record truthfully. I guarantee you, if you do this honestly, you are going to be shocked. We tend to eat *way* more than we think.

We think that if something says it is low fat or low in calories, that it is a 'safe' food. True, and not true. If you eat the serving size the packaging tells you, then you are in the good zone, but, how often have you seen the packaging say 'low calorie' but, not only does it have less calories than the 'normal' one, but it is also *way* smaller. Well, DUH! Of course it will have less calories . . . It's the same size of *half* of the other 'higher' calorie selection. So, when you want to eat it, you tend to eat more than one serving, negating the low fat/low calorie benefit. CHECK THE AMOUNT AND CHECK THE CALORIES!

You also need to wear a pedometer and not walk more than you normally walk. When I first started this experience, I worked an 'on-the-phone' job . . . I wonder why! At the end of my normal eating/ movements (no way to call it *exercising!*) day, I had only walked 687 steps! Ummm . . . and I wondered why I didn't lose weight?

You have now officially been REALITY CHECKED!

*The best *and* worst part of this experience is **DAY 3**. This is the day that you are going to give yourself one and a half hours to eat *any* and *every* food, in any quantity—no calorie documentation *at all*—that you want or think you are going to miss. Word of warning: raw cookie dough and California rolls, bad combination! Pepperoni pizza and chocolate milk . . . a TOTAL science experiment.

Be sure to time yourself. After that hour and a half of eating, without fail, GET RID of any food left. As much as you may feel you have no more room, amazingly, we always find more room when the food is in front of us. Don't think just putting it away is good enough. We have supersensitive hearing and can hear it calling to us. IT MUST LEAVE YOUR HOME!!!

"Now, Lyssa, how in the world is eating everything and anything I want and not having to count calories at all the WORST part???" But . . . wait for it . . . here it comes . . . Oh yeah, here it is: The *guilt*, the *shame*, the *desire to throw up*, and look, they brought along some of their friends, *lowered self-esteem, self-disgust, and self-loathing*. WELCOME!

The result of this hour of binging is to bring about, to put in your face, all the feelings we feel on a large scale each day. In the designated area of your journal, enter exactly how you feel, physically, emotionally, mentally. Sometimes it is hard to find the words, but, again, be honest with yourself. You'll see what you've been feeling all along. Feel it, own it, cry, be ANGRY, be FRUSTRATED, YELL!!!

Okay . . . Now, what are you going to do about it?

(As always, if your doctor has instructed you NOT to eat certain foods, don't eat them. Check with your doctor before beginning any program.)

*Pick a few choice words that really express how you feel. Write them on a small, card-sized paper titled: *Do you really want to do this?* Put it in your wallet in the see-through slot where people normally put their license. Having trouble making a healthy choice when out with friends? Read this. It's not me telling you what to do. It's not some doctor telling you what to do. It is YOUR CHOICE. It's your life. If you like feeling the way you stated on your card, well, go for it. YOU create your life. YOU live your life. YOU choose.

*On another card-sized paper, write a few words of how you will feel when you succeed. Put this in your wallet as well. Some are motivated by the negative of what is. Some are motivated by the positive of what can be. Let's hedge our bets and do both!

My list included being able to buy clothes that didn't have an (or some) X's on the label. Or not having to buy my coat from the men's section. Being able to buy non-stretch jeans, not choking on my chin when I lay on my back, no more snoring . . .

DISGUSTING FAILURE

UNDESIRABLE

UNWORTHY

UGLY

UNLOVABLE

BEAUTIFUL

SUCCESSFUL

TRIUMPHANT

LOVABLE

*Your first weigh-in should be the morning after your huge meal. Do not let this discourage you! You are going to be weighing yourself every day. I can tell you not to become obsessed with a number, but, really, that is pointless to say. I mean, well, isn't the entire reason we are doing this experience to make that number go down? Yes, and then some. We not only want the number on the scale to go down, but the measurements as well, and the clothes size, and the way we feel, and . . .

On this day you will take measurements as well. Make sure that each time you measure; it is in the same spots. Remember, muscle weighs more than fat. Even if your number on the scale isn't lower but the numbers in your measurements are, you win. You are looking better, and, well, isn't that the goal? Let's stick with our theme of honesty. It's great that losing weight will make us healthier, but looking good, feeling confident . . . um, yeah.

*Weigh once a day at the same time in the same place, in the exact same clothes, if you are unable to do it naked. I couldn't weigh naked when I was doing this because I was doing it with four friends. I decided to be kind to them.

WEIGHING IN THE SAME CLOTHES DOES MATTER. DO NOT WEIGH YOURSELF MORE THAN ONCE A DAY! Our weight goes up and down throughout the day. Like any good science project you did in elementary school, you need to have the constant.

When I first started my experience, I had the hardest time following this rule. Especially when I went to the *big* bathroom. I just knew that there was *no way* to weigh the same after as you did before if you had just, well, 'released'. Set a specific time, preferably before you have any food or drink intake and **stick with it**. (P.S. the difference after is more visible on the belly than on the scale, anyway!)

*Guys: disregard the following tip, unless you are doing this experience with your wife.

Reminder: The average woman can gain four to eight pounds of bloat weight while PMSing. This sucks. Not only that, clothes get tighter, you feel puffy, *and* there is a tendency for mood swings and food cravings. Yea! Keep track of your cycle and *try* to remember that when you are PMSing, it may wreak havoc on your scale (read: determination and frustration!) DO NOT let this discourage you. But look! There is a silver lining! If you keep pushing yourself and do what you KNOW you need to do, when the time is over and all that bloating goes away, WOW! You have suddenly lost a TON of weight! Be strong, my sisters, be strong!

Humor will help you through this time. My sister and I liked to imagine our own bumper stickers, for our backsides, not our cars. One of the funniest ones we came up with was:

Something I ate made me swell . . .

Life . . . you gotta laugh . . .

Humor is important, but there are several things you can do during your red-headed Aunt Flo's visit to help in keeping you from completely sabotaging yourself. Soon you are going to be asked to write a list of things to do instead of aimlessly eating. This is going to be the time to use that! This is also the time that you may want to look into purchasing that cardio-kickboxing DVD. It is a great work out and a *wonderful* way to get out the frustration.

Meditation or deep breathing exercises work to help keep your stress in check. The balloon pop is a miracle worker. Blow up a balloon and, with a marker, write whatever you are frustrated with on there. Once you have quite a few problems blown up, grab them with your hands and pop them. Sounds insane, but really works. (P.S. If your husband or children is one of your frustrations, make sure not to let them see their name on the balloon!) Remember to put all the pieces in the waste basket, bending at the waist is exercise, and it feels good to 'throw away' your frustrations. Whatever it is that you do, be sure to remember that you are PMSing, there's a reason they call it, 'the CURSE' and you *will* succeed!

*Reality check: Even though you may feel like you just woke up one day fat, you didn't. You didn't just gain all your weight overnight, and, it isn't going to come off overnight either.

Make your "ultimate" goal, something that seems to be nearly *impossible*, but also have short term goals along the way that are more achievable. When first starting your journey, make sure to make a *lot* of these types of goals, including some non-number goals, like some kind of exercise, or having the guts to start a dance class, or being able to wear a belt. Celebrate these successes with zeal!

When I first started my weight-loss journey, my first goal was to make it through my first day without messing up my diet. My second goal was to do a diet for three days in a row without messing up. The third was for the scale to move down. I didn't care if it was just by an ounce that it went down, all that mattered is that it showed me that I had started; I was *on my way!* The fourth goal was to see a '2' in front of my number.

They were small, simple goals, but they were something that I could achieve, that I could keep building on to succeed in the long run. With each 'small' success, my confidence in myself, the idea and dream that maybe, just maybe I could succeed, grew stronger. **Little goals are the steps to success!**

When you want to be upstairs, you don't just *want* to be upstairs and suddenly you are there. You don't take it from the first step straight to the top. You take it step by step. You begin with the first step, then onto the next, and the next, and the next, and the next, until finally, you've reached the top. Each time you reach a goal, do the "happy bootie" dance! **Enjoy your success no matter how small it may seem in comparison to your "ultimate" goal. Each step is a step to the top!**

*Take before pictures from EVERY angle. No Face Book angles! Be sure to include profile (from the side), front, back, arms, thighs and face. Be sure to make a notation of from where, and what angle you took the picture so you can replicate that same angle the next time, which will be in two weeks.

When you take these pictures, in the beginning, put them somewhere that you aren't going to see them unless you go out of your way to see them. Looking at yourself, in a view that isn't twisted to hide your flaws is something that is hard to accept in the beginning. These pictures, this evidence of who you won't be for much longer needs to be put out of sight . . . not out of mind though! Putting it in a file on your computer with it dated each time will be an awesome slide show after a few months!

Taking pictures is something, as a large person, you might try to avoid. I am telling you to go against what you normally do. I am repeating to you, DO NOT LOOK TOO LONG AT THESE PICTURES IN THE BEGINNING! It is not going to push you! It will depress you. Wait to look until you notice a larger number lost on the scale and/or measurements!

*Find pictures of yourself when you were at, or close to the weight you are aiming for. If you haven't been there yet, no problem. *This* is the time you do the Face Book photo. You know what I am talking about. Look up, tilt chin, lift camera to a position that someone who is about a foot taller would take the picture from, then click (*this* is why you shouldn't believe someone you meet online looks that way in real life!).

Find a body in a magazine that you aspire to have your body look like. Replace their head with yours. Dream, Dream, Dream. Imagine what it is going to feel like when you are there. Awesome, huh?

I had some pictures I had taken when I was eighteen-years-old as ones I aspired to be back to. I had lost a *lot* of weight when I was working out with my brother who was preparing to return to the military. I jogged and did all the physical training each day, with him barking out orders at me as I debated who should get what in my will! But, as much as I may have hated my brother at the time, by the time he had left for overseas, I had lost fifty-five pounds and was a smokin' hot 154 lbs. senior in high school. Later, there are pictures of me getting larger and larger. One picture has me with a hamburger in my face and all I can think when I see it is, "Put the hamburger down! Step away from the food!"

What hurts the most is I remember when I had lost all the weight, I would say, "I'll never let myself get fat again." I even remember saying, "I didn't go through all that pain of losing weight to allow myself to gain it back! No Way!"

Soon after, I moved away to college. You know the idea of the 'freshman fifteen'? Yeah, well, either I was hard of hearing, or I was an over achiever. I did the 'freshman fifty'! In two years of school, I gained ninety-pounds. Having the pictures are vitally important to your success. Remember where you have been. See where you want to be. Even after you reach your goal weight or size, KEEP TAKING PICTURES EVERY TWO WEEKS! This is a good way to keep track and to catch weight gain before it seems like there is too much to lose!

*Position mirrors where you will get the most views of yourself when walking through your home. Look around right now. How many full-length mirrors do you have? The one you may keep is relegated to the inner side of your closet door that you can pretend doesn't exist as you reach in for your standard black outfit. And why is that? What? If you don't see it, neither will others? Sorry sweetie, it doesn't work that way.

How many times, if you actually *do* use your full-length mirror have you looked at it head on and hated what you saw but, if you kind of looked from an angle with your tummy sucked in so much you can't breathe, you looked somewhat better? So, are you going to try to make sure that people *only* see you from that angle. Forget about talking or eating or drinking or . . . oh yeah, *breathing!*

My sister would look in the mirror, squint her eyes, tilt her head and say, "Yep, this looks okay on me, now how am I going to get everyone else to tilt their head and squint their eyes when they look at me?"

Accept your reality, and then *change it!*

*Make a list of things you can easily do when you get the urge to aimlessly snack. Read, walk, dance, paint, have sex. Honestly, I don't care what it is as long as it is NOT eating aimlessly. DON'T just make the list, DO IT!

Things I can do instead of eating:

- call my sister
- go for a walk
- clean out closet/purse/car
- volunteer at local shelter
- reread the awesome *"It Ain't No Darn Diet"* book

*Making lists

On the topic of lists, I am a perpetual list-maker. I usually attribute it to the fact that I have a *horrible* memory, but in all honesty, I just like marking off what I have completed. It makes me feel accomplished. I don't cross off an item on my list when I have done it, instead, I highlight it. That way I can still see all that I have done.

What's more, I don't just write, 'clean house'. Nope, I can't keep it that simple. Cleaning house could take a *long* time to do, and I would just be crossing off one little thing on my list. As compulsive as it sounds, the night before, I make a list of the small things: wash dishes, put dishes away, sweet floors, mop floors, clean dining room table . . . and so on. Marking each of those off feels way better than just marking off, 'clean house'! It sounds crazy, but I feel *great* when I see a long list of things I have accomplished. Try it. It's amazing how much more you will get done!

Actual list I have made:

* **Wash clothes**
* **Dry clothes**
* **Fold clothes**
* **Put clothes away**
* **Make 'To Do' list for tomorrow**
  (I felt accomplished that day!)
* **Get it done**

I may have learned the word, 'procrastination' when I was in fifth grade, but had mastered the meaning *long* before! Putting off the things I didn't like resulted in doing a half-witted job, or not getting things done at all. Use the lovely list that you create, and put a star next to what is super important to get done that day, whether or not it is something you like, and do those first. I *hate* sit-ups and crunches, so I try to get them done in the morning. So, anything starred is one of the first things I do. When I get the things that I don't like to do done in the morning, no matter what else I do or don't get done, I feel accomplished. Feeling good is our goal. Feel good = eat less. Wow!

*List exactly what you want in yourself, physically, mentally and emotionally. State it as if you are already like that. Imagine what it is going to feel like when you are 'there'. Imagine the feel of your clothes, the feeling of being able to buy an outfit because you like it, not because it is one of the few that fits. Imagine what it is like when weight isn't an issue anymore. Make this a reality. **Imagining you are already there will help you make the right choices when you are faced with daily temptations.** If you already see yourself as thin, would the skinny you order the jumbo fries?

Decisions I would make when I was fat:

* Order a Venti caramel Frapiccino (Regular milk)
* Hold the throw pillow on the couch in my lap while sitting to, ahem, *hide* my belly!
* Celebrate *any* achievement or success with FOOD
* Treat myself to a *lot* of unhealthy food because I deserved it when I had a bad day

Choices I make now I'm skinny:

* Order tea, or at least a *skinny* tall caramel frapiccino
* Not order dessert until *after* I have already eaten my (healthy) meal
* Celebrate my successes with something FUN!

*Let me introduce you to your new frenemies: Girdie the Girdle and Tighty Whitey Tee. WEAR TIGHT CLOTHES WHEN YOU EAT. Ever notice when you go to a buffet you plan what to wear so you can eat as much as you want without being hampered by restrictive clothing? We eat to our clothes consumption. Wear the tighter ones under your normal clothes, if necessary.

As simple as this may sound to be, "Really Lyssa . . . Wear tight clothes? I don't have any of those . . ." We all have at least one shirt that is a second skin. Now is the time you should wear it. Granted, you may not want to wear it on its own, you do want to *feel* it hugging you. This is one time that it needs to stay against your skin.

I am sure you all know the feeling of when you sit down and you just *know* that parts of your shirt are tucked in your rolls so you do the 'shift-pull' as deftly as possible to try to escape the notice of others seeing you *pull material from between the rolls!* Tight clothes make you uncomfortable. Guess what, so does fat! This will help you be aware of how much you eat. CREATE AWARENESS!

* Shout it out Loud

Tell people you are around often that you are trying to lose weight, that you are doing this 'experience,' that you are on a diet. Why, you may ask . . . well, nobody likes to be ashamed. Humans are humans. Remember all the times you have been ashamed of your weight? Remember how it felt? Sucked, huh? We can't change our nature, but we can find a way to use it to our advantage. It is great to tell kids to not worry about what others think of them, but, truth be told, we DO worry what others think of us. Wow! What a great tool for us to use. Think about it. If you tell people in your office or at home, or wherever you are most often at, that you are on a diet and then you are pigging out in front of them, how is that going to look to them? This is a great way for you to use your internal peer pressure to force yourself to push through you cravings, your desire to eat things you know you shouldn't. The best part of it is how they look at you with more respect for being strong, and even better, is the way you feel after you have been strong and held your resolve! **Yea for peer pressure!**

*Clip any motivational stories you find

They don't even have to be about weight loss. People who have succeeded despite the odds don't have some super-human power you don't have. They just found the determination and perseverance we all have somewhere inside us that we have to find ourselves. Some of the people I look up to most actually had a tough time, or *a lot* of tough times in their life. Before, I always thought they must have something special that was absent in me. How horrible is that?!? I mean, imagine if you were these people who worked their behinds off to get where they are in life, who didn't have everything just *handed* to them, and then you have these people like *I* used to be who didn't give them the credit they were due. Augh! How *lazy* was I to make up any excuse for why they could succeed and I couldn't because I didn't want to accept my *blame* of my lot in life! I am so thankful that I never got the chance to meet most of these successful people at that time. I know if I was them, and I knew others assumed that I just 'got lucky' in succeeding despite the odds, or that I was 'in the right place at the right time' . . . Ewww! Yeah, they *were* in the right place at the right time. They were in the right mental place! They consciously made the choice that they were going to do all they could to succeed. "Yeah, but doors were opened for them." Of course doors opened, because *they* turned the knob and pushed! As long as you just keep thinking that they were just lucky or in the right place at the right time, YOU WILL NEVER SUCCEED. **Own up to your responsibility for your life and realize that the ability to change is only from YOU.** Read these motivational stories with the knowledge that one day, someone might be reading about you!

*Cheer Squad

Be your own cheerleader. At the beginning of your experience, family and friends tend to be very supportive of you. They will tell you they support you often and listen to all you 'stories' of what you are doing, eating, the energy you are gaining . . . but, what is interesting to you is not interesting too long to other people. If you are truly embarking on this journey with the idea that you are completely transforming your life, which is a total possibility, it is *the* most important thing to you. Everybody is self-centered; it's called, 'being human,' but sometimes, especially if you have been especially large and especially neglectful of yourself, giving and doing for others way more than you do for yourself, even though they may want what is best for you, sometimes family and friends have a hard time accepting that you are no longer available at any and every moment. It is hard for them to accept. It is hard for them to accept that you are going to be taking time for yourself and the word NO is going to actually come out of your mouth! Usually, they want what is good for you. But, even though you are embarking on this amazing, life-transforming experience, they may not be, and, just like when you go through a tragedy in life that takes time to recuperate from, their support and cheer may only last so long. Then it comes down to you. Enjoy this journey. Feel the good and tell others of the good, of your successes. This will not only help you, it may inspire them! "No man is an island," but sometimes, in your journey, you may feel like you are the only one. That is okay. This is a great way to develop your pep squad of one!

I am strong!

I will begin!

And in the end,

I AM THIN!

Yea, ME!

*Clean, Clean, Clean!

Everybody knows the old saying, "cluttered home, cluttered mind." There's a reason these sayings stay around; they're true. We are *amazing* at making excuses for why we don't have time to keep things clean. Look around your home right now. Take a good look. If someone from your work, church, school . . . *wherever,* came to your door now, would you want to invite them in for coffee? Don't just look at the main entry room. Are you like some who have just the one room clean but, Heaven forbid, they have to use the restroom! Or you have to make sure to close all the doors to the other rooms that are not so 'presentable.' Or, if they follow you into the kitchen as you go to make the coffee and you are trying to delay them, mentally willing them to go sit down! Yeah, I have *no idea* what that is like!

What I did realize is that my home was like my body; a big mess! Just like my weight gain was a result, and not the problem, it is the same for my home. It is almost as if I just gave up on life. I wasn't alive, I was just going through the motions. This experience is not just about losing weight, it is about taking control. Like the title says, this is NOT a diet! This is not about just changing what you eat; this is about changing your life. Remember the times when you were a kid that your parents would make you clean your room after your closet had a bout of bulimia? Remember how good it felt to sit in you room when it was clean? I would want all my friends to come over just to *see* my clean room. Yeah, imagine that on a larger scale with your home. You cannot take control of your life if you cannot take control of your home. Blast your music, dance while cleaning. Guess what! THAT'S exercise! Cleaning is one of the few things in life that we can see instantaneous results. Go. Clean. Now!

*Get organized

This, of course, goes along with the cleaning, but, okay. Let's think about it. I'm asking you to give yourself an extra ten minutes in the morning to start your day off great. Where are you going to get those ten minutes? Last time I checked, I'm pretty sure there's still just twenty-four hours in the day, no matter how many times you may have wished for more. Until we find a way to make more than twenty-four hours in the day, you are going to have to figure out how to get done what needs to be done in the time you have.

Time is the one thing we cannot create, but can definitely waste! It is the one thing we cannot purchase when there isn't any left, and no one can give back to you once it is gone. One of the biggest arguments we hear is that there just isn't enough time to exercise or cook healthy or, or, or . . . Okay, I get it. Life is busy. ORGANIZE and PRIORITIZE!

When you get mail, open it immediately. Put a file or tray for the things that have to be taken care of immediately. Have a recycling bin for the things that aren't important. Have another tray for things you may want to look into more later on. A push-pin board is great for having a calendar marked with the dates bills are due, sticky-notes of important reminders (color coded) and a place to tack the bills that need to be paid soon. It *will* take some time to create this, but in the end, the time saved looking for papers, and money saved from not having the late fees tacked on will allow for you to have more time for YOU and less stress! Double whammy! Awesome!

Get your clothes out for the week on Sunday. This includes socks, underwear, making sure your pantyhose don't have a run . . . Oh, wow! You've just found some time. Put a bowl or hook by the door for your keys. Oh yeah! Lookie there . . . MORE time found!

If you have not worn a particular pair of shoes in at least a year, ladies, I'm talking to you, GET RID OF THEM! And, if by some freak of nature, you have clothes that are *already* too big for you, well, why in the world would you keep them? Are you PLANNING on getting fatter? *Exactly* . . . GET. RID. OF. THEM!

Use your time wisely!

*Get a friend to try these new experiences with you

Be careful who you choose. Beware! Misery loves company, and if you choose someone who quits easily or doesn't want to push hard, well, they may try to guilt you into staying back with them. It is hard enough to push yourself, but when someone else is slacking off, it is all the easier to excuse yourself.

As a fat chick, I know we tend to be friends with other fat chicks. They "get" us. Problems occur when one of the herd decides to change their life and the others haven't made that same decision. Envy, jealousy, shame for not pushing themselves, fear of losing their binging buddy, whatever the reason, they may subconsciously (or consciously) try to sabotage your success. As hard as it may be to realize, a true friend is supportive. If they aren't supportive, they aren't your friend—Plain and simple.

I had one friend that I began my experience with years ago. We had been friends from school and had gone through all the times of being made fun of together. We both knew what it was like growing up fat, and when I started this experience, I thought she would be the one person who would understand the most, who would be the most supportive. I was wrong. She wasn't ready.

It wasn't that she didn't want me to succeed, but because she wasn't ready, it was hard for her to accept my attempt at changing my life. I learned early on in my experience to not tell her of frustrations or any of the, ech, weight gains or my times of 'failure'. If I ever complained, she would remind me of all the excuses I had given myself before of why I was just 'meant' to be fat. I already had that voice in my head. I didn't need her voice as well. We are still friends, but, unfortunately, not like we once were.

This experience is great, but not easy. It isn't just the diet and exercise that is going to be difficult, but your entire life is going to be affected. There are going to be hard decisions, beyond the decision of eating the doughnut or not. You have to be strong and choose wisely who you have join you. Sometimes you may lose more than just weight. This is something you need to understand from the beginning.

*Be around positive people

This might not be something you can always control, but, at least do your best to refrain from being around negative people. Have you ever noticed how, you could be having a great day, and at the end of your day you call your friend and she goes on and on about how bad her day or life is? And, ridiculously, the more they go on talking about all their negatives, not only do you feel like you would be an insensitive jerk by saying how great your day was, but you try *empathizing* with them. You feel if you tell them any of your achievements that it is as if you are saying, "Hey, I know your life totally sucks right now but let me tell you how fabulous mine is!" Suddenly, we find ourselves *trying* to find bad things that happened in our day. Then, if we can't find something bad in THAT day, we resort to bad times past, and bring up those and all the negative feelings that come with them. Are you

KIDDING me? Come on! Life is short. Enjoy the good. If a friend is bringing you down and, of course you are a good friend and want to help them up, but, DO NOT let them hinder your success. Do not let them do the whole 'drowning person/life guard thing'. You know what I'm talking about. I'm sure you heard stories of when a lifeguard's trying to save a drowning person and is drowned by the person they are trying to save.

Some people are just natural whiners. They will sit and complain about the unfairness of life, yet not lift a finger to change it. Some people are complainers. These point out things they are not happy with and then, get this; they *do* something to change it! Wow! Life is never perfect, for anybody, but if your friend is a complainer, not a whiner, this is good. If they just want to moan and *whine*, suddenly have something you need to do and let them drown someone else. Seems selfish, I know, but, sometimes you have to think of yourself to succeed.

*Dress well!

Have you ever noticed the bigger the size, the bigger the flowers? STOP! We do not want to look like a flippin' rose garden! We tend to wear the one-size-fits-all, as in a whole *lot*, you know, those lovely shirts or dresses with the ties in the back to loosen or tighten, according to your body's need. Ties are for trash bags. Women, I know you could go to your closet right now and find *at least* three of these tops. I would bet that not only do they have the hefty, hefty, cinch ties, but they also have a very low 'v neck' that shows the joining of the twins, and a flow of material beneath them. Fine. Keep them . . . for now, but ASAP, get rid of them. Wearing a tent does not disguise the fact that you are big.

Stop with the moo-moos. You're not fooling anyone. What? You want to make sure you're ready if you have to suddenly visit Hawaii? Really? No, you're not a size four, but you also are not a sofa. Leave the tents for camping.

I'm not saying to wear something that shows everything, but there ARE some nice things out there, thankfully. The other day I saw plus-size mannequins! I'm not saying that we should all stay large, but it is great to see that there are nice things we can wear while we are here.

*On what to wear

Yes, we want to feel sexy, regardless of our size, but, have you noticed that there are a lot of livin' large women who show a TON of boobage? It screams, "Look here, look here! Just don't look any further!" A hint of cleavage is sexy. Looking as if you could just lean to the left and out pops a milkshake maker . . . NOT sexy. As I wish for any woman of ANY size, HAVE SELF RESPECT and dress to show it.

*On the subject of clothes

I'll admit, when I first started going to the gym, I wore TERRIBLE clothes. I wanted to wear the biggest shirt I could because, when I was on the stationary bike and each time my knee come up my stomach was pushed up, pushing my chest up into the lovely folds of my chin, there is the idea that, no matter what I wore, I was going to look bad.

I was more concerned with being able to wear something that I could walk without rubbing my thighs raw or having the 'A line" shorts; you know, when the friction of your thighs rubbing together lead to the inside of your 'cool-lots' (which are so not "cool") bunching up at the top. I also had to worry about the same raw effect that happened between my thighs also happening from the fat of my arms rubbing against the side of my chest. When you are so large, there doesn't seem to be any clothes that are 'comfortable,' rather, you look for what is the least '*un*comfortable.'

Rule of thumb: tight legging and tight, long-sleeve shirts below whatever you are wearing is hot, but a total skin saver! That way you don't have to jog (walk with a bounce) with your elbows in the air!

Once I figured out the tighter underclothes, I just put whatever was loose on top. I didn't care if it was stained, mismatching, torn in some places. I figured it didn't matter because, well, when you are over three-hundred pounds of flesh shaking on the Stair Master, did it really matter what it was covered with?

Answer: Yes. Not only was I showing others I had low self-esteem by not caring what I looked like, I only re-enforced it to myself. After I lost my first twenty pounds, yeah, I was still in the 280's, I went and bought a matching gym outfit. I wasn't blind. I knew I wasn't hot sexiness, but I did look like I cared about myself. Crazily enough, it made a *huge* difference.

*On the subject of clothes, and the departure of some

If you had looked in my closet a few years ago, you would think I was sharing that storage space with a few different people. In a way, I was. I had fat clothes, medium clothes, skinny clothes, stretch clothes, non-stretch . . . The sizes ranged from a seven (yeah, that was a *while* ago!) to a 24. And those 24's were stretch! I had yo-yo dieted and gained and lost most of my life, that I was afraid to get rid of *anything*. I didn't want to get rid of the smaller because, hey, I'm going to get there one day, and I didn't want to get rid of the larger because, oh crap, I might be there again one day . . . Okay, let's think about it. If I have clothes from when I was, *amazingly*, thin, and I am able to fit into them again, well, it was about twelve years ago that I was that size. I'm pretty sure the style has changed. If there is a favorite, keep it and ditch the rest. As for the larger clothes, well that's all sorts of wrong keeping them. I was afraid of my failure. I had failed so many times before, I was just planning and preparing myself for the next failure. I really hope I don't have to explain how that is wrong.

Really? I do. Okay. Well, if you *prepare* to fail, *you are going to fail.* If you have a 'plan B,' your bigger clothes, 'plan A', *not needing your bigger clothes,* will fail. Got it? Good.

So, as you lose weight and something becomes too big for you, you have one of two choices. Either, say it with me here, GET RID OF IT, or, get it tailored immediately. Are you planning to gain weight back? Are you planning to fail? Keeping those clothes is giving yourself permission to go back. BURN THAT BRIDGE! That is not a path you want to choose to walk again!

Doubting your resolve? Do you like being insecure? Do you like feeling like the hippo in the zoo being watched as you grocery shop? Set your resolve to succeed. Give yourself no choice. "Screw-it, I have to keep losing. I got rid of all my fat clothes."

*DO, DO, DO!

Do keep one pair of pants (NOT your stretchy pants!) that you wore in the beginning. Seeing the number difference on the scale is great, but being able to hold your new "skinny" jeans in front of the old and seeing the difference is way more amazing! Besides, when you reach your goal, you have to do your whole infomercial picture with your old jeans on as you hold out the waist to show the weight loss. Just be sure you are NEVER wearing these pants again!

This is a crazy idea, and I so wish I had done it, but, record your inspirational infomercial now, before you have lost your weight. Make a script. What are you going to say? Pretend you have already lost all the weight. Who do you think you would inspire? This will help you; to visualize your success. This is a great way to put positive pressure on yourself to succeed. How awesome is it going to be to make that *exact* same commercial when you actually have reached your goal? How cool is that going to be?!?

*Back to the lists

Make a list of people you admire, people you would like to be like. Why do you admire them? What *exactly* is it about them that makes them admirable? Is it their strength, their kindness, their ability to make a difference? What do they have that makes them a success? Do you notice certain aspects of each, that they all have in common?

I admire a lot of people. I don't like them all, but I admire certain aspects of them. I respect the way Angelina Jolie helps the less fortunate (and she's really hot!), I admire Hillary Clinton's ability to remain stoic in public while dealing with something that should have been a private humiliation. I admire Oprah (who doesn't), for her openness, her willingness to allow the public to know her past, as painful as it may be. My list goes on and on.

What do these people have in common? What is it they have that I don't? How do they overcome what brings many to their knees? Aspire to find what it is about these people you admire, find these same strengths within yourself and then build on them!

*Practice NOW who you want to become

Famous people aren't our only examples of who or how we want to become. We all know those people we see who appear to naturally exude all of those traits you want to have. They sit the right way, smile perfectly, and seem to have practiced every movement they make. They look so graceful. They always seem poised and in control.

When I lost the first one-hundred pounds, it took me a long time to realize I was no longer that three-hundred-pound monster. I didn't realize that it wasn't just my weight I had to work on, but all the negatives that came along with it.

Look around. No, REALLY look around. Observe how larger people stand, sit, walk. Now observe how thin people walk, sit and stand. There . . . you see it? Do you see the difference?

Notice the way larger people tend to walk with their toes pointed slightly to the side as if to better support the shifting of their weight. Notice how larger people tend to walk and stand with their palms facing behind them.

Look how people sit. Where are their legs? Women: practice crossing your legs in your home! Make sure you are able to do it all the way before you start crossing your legs in public. No woman looks sexy with her ankle on top of her knee. Oh, and be careful of tables! I have knocked over a ton of drinks when attempting to cross my legs under tables! Oh my, so *not sexy*!

Look at arm placement. Unless you are mad and wanting the person to know you are angry, *do not* cross your arms across your chest. That's all we need to do, add more girth to our ... well, girth! And word-to-the-wise: if you are going to be carrying two drinks, DO NOT THINK HOLDING THEM IN FRONT OF YOUR STOMACH IS GOING TO HIDE IT! Hold them up and on either side of the "twins." Wow! Look at that frame you create, shifting the eyes away from the DANGER zone! WORK ON THIS NOW! Make it a habit. Just the loss of a ton of weight isn't going to change your life, YOU have to make a conscious effort to do that. Begin now making those changes!

*Put yourself first

If you have ever paid attention to the flight attendant on the plane as they go over the safety instructions, they give you the *best* advice! They inform you that, in the event of an emergency, oxygen masks will drop down. If you are a mother, the natural instinct is to help your child first. But, we are instructed to put our own mask on FIRST before assisting others. I asked an attendant why a mother would put hers on before her child and the attendant responded, "Well, the mother is no help to her child if she has fainted." BRILLIANT!

We are no good to the rest of the world, our children, our spouses, our bosses, or our friends, if we are not taking care of ourselves first. Think of a water bottle. You can only pour so much out without refilling. Before you have nothing left to give, realize **you need to refill**.

Stop being a flippin' martyr! You are either one of these people, or you know one. You know who you are. Martyrs are the ones that won't put on make-up because they like for others to see just how tired or rushed they are; picking the kids up from school in the sexy baggy sweats and their husband's t-shirt from some chili cook-off. They, or *you,* are the one who, when someone offers help, sigh a long, weary, 'I'm carrying the weight of the world,' sigh and say, 'Oh, I couldn't bother you. I can take care of this.'

Really . . . get over yourself. Get over your pride, your desire to have a complaint-worthy life and learn to accept help. Say no to taking on more than you should, and do something just for you.

Moral of the story: Take care of yourself. There is no reason to feel guilty for taking care of you.

*BE HAPPY ALREADY!

Stop saying, "I'll be happy when . . ." Be happy now. Even if you haven't lost a single ounce, you are taking the first step in taking control of your life. "What do you mean, Lyssa?" Well, you're reading this book, aren't you? Appreciate the small victories along the way. 'Woo Hoo! I said no to the doughnut today! I ROCK!' If you don't appreciate it, you'll never keep it.

Have you ever been in such a bad mood that even *you* wished you could get away from yourself? It is hard when life is difficult to stay happy, or upbeat, or, well, at least not getting depressed as heck! But, you have to make that choice. You can be sad and down, but, really, where is that going to get you? How often do you see someone with a scowl on their face and think, "Hey, that looks like a fun guy! Let me go get to know him!" Look in the mirror right now. Are you that? Are you someone you would want to get to know, or are you the one that sucks the happiness out of a room? Check yourself. Fix yourself! Be aware of your facial expressions. So, yeah, smile . . .

*SMILE!

Oooo! Like the segway? Anyway, as simple as it may sound, smile, smile smile! "Really, Lyssa . . . This will help me lose weight?" Yes, siree, it will.

Smiling not only helps you, but it's true that it is contagious. Even if the contagion is just the fact that people feel obligated to return a smile, real or not! When you smile, real or not, it releases serotonin, you know, the happy hormone. Even if you are fake-smiling, you fool your brain and suddenly, you actually begin to feel happier. Feeling happier leads to less eating out of anger or sadness. Smiling—a free gastric bypass!

Look there! Not only are you helping yourself, you are changing the world, one smile, one person at a time; making your day, and day of others, happy. Wow! What a kind, selfless person you are! Celebrate your greatness!

*On the subject of faking it

I used to think that successful people were just born to be that way. Okay, maybe for some, this is the case. Growing up, being fat most of the time, I had a lot of free time on my hands, and not a lot of friends. I had a lot of time to observe, and one thing I noticed is, when people, even the successful or popular people, think nobody is watching, you can see a bit of their insecurity. If you watch closely, you will see that they have their own ideas of what isn't good enough about them.

Because of all my observations from my invisible years (yeah, when you are fat, you are either stared at or invisible), I have become a strong believer of, "Fake it 'til you make it." There are so many books out there on this topic. Uh, isn't that merely positive thinking, believing leading to achieving, "putting the power out there?" Read these books. Follow what works for you. Whatever it is that makes your life better, run with it.

Humans can be clever, but also manipulated as well. People will often perceive you as who you present yourself to be. Don't sell yourself short. A way to put this in perspective for you: Pretend you are introducing your child to a group of people. Are you going to say, "Please say hello to my heifer of a daughter. She is so not worthy of you even speaking to her, but please take pity on her and be her friend. Please, oh please be her friend! Don't worry, she will allow you to walk all over her because she knows she is nothing and should just be so grateful for you to allow her to be in your presence." Um, yeah . . . I would love to say this is something that is just created from my mind, but looking back, that is how I presented myself to people. I didn't literally say *those* words, but I may as well have!

Present yourself as you would present your daughter. Present yourself as the 'dream you' and watch your dream become a reality.

Now, don't get me wrong. If you are as big as I was, you aren't going to wave your imagination wand and make them see Victoria Beckham when they look at you, but you can make it so they see *you,* not just your outside.

*Run with the compliment

I am SOOO sick of giving someone a compliment about something good they are wearing or how their hair looks, and hearing back, "this old thing" or "it would be better if I wasn't so fat!" or "yeah, yeah . . ."

Augh! Take a freakin' compliment and let it make you feel good. How do you feel when people do that to you? Does it make *you* feel good? When someone compliments you and you respond negatively, such as above, you not only negate what could be a total bonus for you, you make the person who complimented you feel like crap, and totally rethink the whole idea of ever saying something good about you again.

I will say it time and time again. We are human. As humans, we need to hear good things about ourselves. We have no problem telling children good things about themselves to make them have a better self-esteem, but that seems to happen less and less the older we get. Just because we are adults doesn't mean that we don't need some of the same ego stroking. That said, when we do get that compliment we so crave, don't negate it!

When someone says something nice to you, or compliments you, when you respond as mentioned before, how do you think the person who complimented you is going to feel? What do you think *they* are going to think. Well, even if they don't say it out loud, their thought process could be as following:

"Gee, thanks . . . I'll be sure not to compliment you again!"

Then you have lost the chance of not only making you feel better, you have just released a whole lot of negative at them. Good job!

A simple, "Thank you! You made my day." Or just "Thank you!" with a smile is the perfect answer. If someone compliments you on your weight loss, DO NOT SAY, "Oh, but I have so much more to go."

Just say thank you and feel the glory of your success.

*Aim for "slut"

No, don't sleep around—hello?-DISEASES!

If you are working this hard to make your body look good, a man, or woman (your choice) should have to work just as hard to get it!

A few weeks ago I borrowed a shirt from my sister. It fit really well and I loved how it looked. Of course I did what came naturally; I showed it off to my sister. The first words that came out of her mouth were, "You slut!"

It wasn't that the shirt was skimpy or anything, but the two of us know exactly what she meant. When I was larger, *much* larger, when we were out and saw a hot chic, we would look at each other and say, 'slut.' I know, I know, what mean, jealous people we were. But, can you honestly say you have never said or thought the same?

We all know the root of this reaction is the lovely green-eyed monster, but, there is a little monster in all of us if we admit it. How many times have you been out, and you have dressed the best that you can, just to see someone who looks like she rolled out of bed gorgeous. First, it is *rare* anybody wakes up sexy, and secondly, instead of looking at her and having the gut reaction of jealousy, imagine what it is like to be her. Imagine what a day in her life is like, even down to what she eats. What is it about her that makes her someone you would envy? What are her mannerisms? What is her body language?

Know that if you stick to your experience, you too, will one day be called a "slut." Congratulations!

S—super
L—looking
U—u want to be like
T—type

*You HAVE to make time to exercise

Period. If you can't take a big block of time, find ten minutes at least three times a day. This is great for the metabolism and is just as effective. NO EXCUSES!

This goes back to doing things for yourself. You doing this experience is not only going to help you, it will put you in a better position to help others. There are numerous benefits to benefits to exercising. Most importantly, it makes you less flabby!

I know, I know, there are a million reasons you can't get to exercising:

* I need to clean
  - Uh . . . cleaning *is* exercising!

* The time it takes to get dressed, to the gym, and showered afterwards just takes too much time out of my day
  - Don't you normally shower everyday anyway?
  - Oh yeah, you could work out at home!

* **The gym is too crowded at this time**
  - What great motivation to push yourself harder!

* I promised my in-laws I'd go visit
  - Wow, really stretching it there, huh?

* I just want to finish this television show I started watching
  - So, it's better to watch people pretending to live a life than going out and living your own?

* I'm gonna be sore tomorrow if I do . . .
  - Uh, duh. No pain, all weight gain!

I am giving you the tricks to find more time in your day, but you are the one who has to find the motivation and determination to do the right thing with that extra time.

*Play time!

There seems to be an epidemic of children being obese. Why is that? Could it be because computers, televisions, and all other sorts of electronics are being used as babysitters? Could it be that we have made our lives so busy that we don't have time to stop and enjoy the simple fun of what it is to be a child?

As an aunt of amazing nieces and nephews, play time is my all-time favorite time. How often do we get the chance to act like a kid? Sometimes I take my nieces or nephews to the park to play; not so *they* can play, but so that *I* can play. Think about it, a thirty-one-year-old woman playing in a kid's park by herself . . . *creepy!*

I agree. There are times that we need to be able to sit with other moms and actually have 'adult talk'. That is totally understandable. So, make time for that, but don't forget to make time for your kids. Show them that they are not your burden, rather they are your blessing.

Don't just take your kids to the park, or tell them to go play outside, and then sit and watch from the sidelines as you are trying to accomplish a million other things at once. Life is not a spectator sport! Join in on the fun. Savor each moment. Life is a conglomeration of moments, and this moment will be gone momentarily. Don't miss it. One day you will turn around and they won't need you anymore. Don't miss their fun years because you are so busy doing something else. Teach them the games you used to play. Remember hop-scotch? Red-Rover? Remember how good it felt when your parents paid full attention to you? Pass that on to your child.

There are so many benefits to this suggestion. You and your child get to have great, quality time together *and* you are getting exercise! Just because you can't measure the calories doesn't mean you aren't burning them!

*Gym Shoes

This is to negate a possible excuse you have up your sleeve. 'Oh, I would absolutely *love* to be able to take a quick walk during lunch, but, I just can't in these heels!'

Keep a pair of gym shoes in the trunk of your car. You never know when you are going to get an extra ten to fifteen minutes, such as the end of your lunch break. Wow! What a great chance to take a quick stroll. As much as walking around the block in high-heels may look sexy and majorly work your calves, blisters on the balls of your feet . . . not so sexy. Be sure to have a clean pair of socks. If you are wearing panty hose, women, this is for you, you know how stinky that can be if you sweat in your shoes! The best idea is to keep your gym bag in your car. That way you have all the necessary supplies available to return to your work revitalized and refreshed. There are a few supplies that are a must:

- shoes
- socks
- brush
- powder
- deodorant

- water
- perfume
- work out pants

The pants are great to have, especially if they are tighter to put under your skirt, again, ladies, this is for you! You don't want to return to work looking like you just got out of the gym. Make sure to keep your exercise necessities in your trunk so you never miss an opportunity.

By the way, a walk in the middle of a stressful day is a great way to clear the mind and create a sense of peace so that when you return back to work, you are able to find resolutions to any problem that may arrive. Wow, exercising *and* improving your ability at work. Another double bonus!

*Parking

While we are on the subject of sneaking exercise into our work day . . . Work is stressful, and sometimes we are bombarded with issues the moment we enter our office. If you have ever woken up late, quickly dressed, ate breakfast on the drive to work and walked into work still feeling half asleep, you know your thinking and problem resolution skills are not at peak performance.

As a teacher, the moment I stepped on the school ground, I had to be in teacher mode. It didn't matter whether or not it had a good night's sleep. I didn't matter if I was completely *exhausted.* I had

Melissa Mathis

to suck it up and fake enthusiasm I *definitely* wasn't feeling at 7:30 in the morning! A trick I learned was one that I had heard many times before. Park further away. Yep, that's it.

I have never understood why people who are going to the gym to work out and burn calories wait forever for a closer parking spot. Uh, hello? Aren't you going to the gym to exercise? Last time I checked, walking IS exercise. It goes for anywhere you have to park. With that extra time you keep finding in the day, try leaving a little earlier so you can park a bit farther from the door for the extra walking. You get that extra bit of exercise, *and* you get that little extra boost of energy!

Same goes for elevators verses stairs. Now, if you work on the tenth floor and are just beginning the whole work out idea, it might not be the best idea to do the whole ten flights, but, do the first four then grab an elevator the rest of the way. The rest of the ride up will give you time to stop huffing and puffing . . . we are aiming for extra energy, not an asthma attack as you're walking into the office! What a great way to get a bit of extra exercise, get your heart rate up, and rev your body and mind for the day of work.

64

*Exercise is great, any exercise

There are so many different types of exercises out there. I love to go to the gym because, once you are there, there really is no other option than to work out. When I can't make it to the gym, or am feeling too lazy to go, I pop in a dvd. Hip Hop Abs is amazing, working out the stomach without lying on my back, Rock on! The belly dancing ones are fun, even with my lack of coordination and all.

Regardless of which exercise you choose, enjoy it. If you don't like one, try another. What's important is to exercise, period.

Just remember to try to leave two hours from when you complete the exercise to when you sleep. Right after a workout, I would be exhausted, but give me an hour and it feels as if I had drunk three cups of coffee.

If time leaves you no choice in the matter, ALWAYS opt to exercise!

*Gyms

If you have never seen the inside of a gym, other than those on television, choosing one can be difficult.

Look for one that is close to home: If you have to drive too far, well, that is just another potential excuse to not go. Finding one the opposite direction of rush hour traffic is ideal. Don't expect to feel a hundred percent comfortable when you first walk in, but it has to have a comfortable enough atmosphere that you will go. Most, if not all, gyms will give a free pass so you can test it out and see if you want to join. Use this! It is a great way to see if it is for you!

If the commercial for a gym showed a bunch of women on the Stair Master with a smile on their lips and a thong in their cheeks, more than likely my three-hundred pound 'thong-maker of full-butt panties' bootie was not going to be comfortable there. Choose wisely. If you join a gym because you think you are going to look like the people in their commercials, but you are too insecure in your sweats and tent—tee to go, then you are just losing money and losing time.

*Ambition

How many times have you been overly ambitious and say, "I am going to wake up forty-five minutes early and jog/do an aerobics video/work out . . ." and then hit snooze five times that morning and feel like a failure. How about giving yourself just ten minutes extra in the morning? You can use these ten minutes to stretch, do yoga, jog in place, or say your 'I ams' (The 'I ams' will be explained a bit later in this book). Plan to wake up ten minutes earlier . . . and succeed! We are all about small steps. There is a chance that your ten minutes may one day turn into twenty. Some people may be born naturally ambitious, but if that isn't you, you need to find it. You need to reach inside and pull it out of you!

*Pick your exercise

Beware of doing something that is going to bulk you up, unless that is what you want, but, at 300, I figure I was "bulked" enough. Zumba, or any other dancing, the elliptical machine . . . these are great aerobic exercises to burn calories without building too many bulky muscles.

As a big woman, aerobic exercise WAS anaerobic (muscle building) as well! You try dancing with all that weight on you and tell me it's not. Yeah, the pros are right; the more muscle you have, the more calories you will burn. But, especially in the beginning, you are going to build a lot of muscle anyway because you have your very own built in barbells! Besides, if you are looking to see a smaller number on the scale, remember muscle weighs more than fat and it is hard to get that through our heads, no matter how smart we are. Until you are able to get that, aerobic is the way to go. Swimming and walking are great for this.

*Try different classes

Don't' get bored. Just like your diet, if you keep doing the same thing every day, you are going to get bored. Try new things, even if you have *no* idea how to do it. Mix it up. Zumba and hip hop dance are great for having fun and burning calories. AND, you are so busy trying to learn the steps without making a fool of yourself; you don't realize YOU ARE EXERCISING!

Body combat and cardio kickboxing are great after a frustrating day at work. My sister loves step aerobics, but, even 'til today, I suck at it. By the time I figure out how to do the 'twirly bird' the rest of the class has moved on and I'm about four other exercises behind.

Try each class, sport or equipment at least twice. The first time could be a fluke. It took me about three months for me to be able to understand the basic steps. Keep pushing yourself. The goal is, if you are not someone who looks forward to the gym, at least you don't want to despise it! Never be afraid of being the only one who doesn't know the moves or isn't able to keep up. Just walk in (to the back), smile, and do your best while learning to laugh at yourself.

*Maximize your workouts

If you are anything like me, you want to make sure that you get the most results from the least amount of effort. I think that is everybody's goal. One of the first rules to remember is to not do the exact exercise, except for swimming, for more than fifteen minutes straight.

The elliptical machine is one of my favorite exercise machines because it is the one I have found that burns the most amount of calories the soonest and doesn't kill my knees. As much as I love watching the calories accrue, after fifteen minutes your muscles become efficient to that particular exercise, and work less, burning less. One trick to do is, after fifteen minutes, switch directions—forward to backward, backward to forward. You will get tired, and bored. Switch to different machines if necessary then come back to the original one. Keep moving, and keep on going!

*Wear a pedometer

The more steps you take, the better. Just think of each step as a step away from the things that hurt you; the life you don't like. Wearing a pedometer is especially great for the first two days of this experience when you are eating how you normally eat. Don't walk anymore in those first days than you normally would. Record how many steps you take. Way less than you expected, huh? Every day is going to be a different amount depending on what you do that day. We tend to walk *way* less than the generations before us.

Be sure not to cheat when you are recording! Before you get in the car, check how many steps are recorded. Check again when you get out of the car. Sometimes it may record more steps from the vibrations. Subtract the extra. DO NOT LIE TO YOURSELF!

There are many ways that you can make walking more effective. When I was looking for new work out dvd's I was surprised to see one for walking. How is a dvd going to teach us to do something we learned when we were toddlers? Shockingly, there are actually a ton of things you can do to burn more calories while walking.

One way is to alternate the speed at which you walk. Sounds simple, but is frustrating to do sometimes. If you speed walk for five minutes, then shuffle for one minute (as if you are wearing the cuffs they put on prisoners feet), and then stroll for two minutes. Then repeat. The whole point seems to keep your heart from expecting what's coming next.

Another way you can make it more effective is to use walking sticks. These are the ones that look like ski poles that you use like the sticks people use when they are hiking. This is great to add to get a great arm work out as well!

Arm weights. These are great, but don't put them around your ankles. Long term use of ones around the ankle may harm your ankle.

Aim for 10,000 steps a day. Sounds like a lot, and after measuring the amount you walk on a 'normal' day, it may seem downright impossible. Make it possible. Find the extra steps in your day!

*Yoga/stretching . . . brilliant!

When I was first working out, I was told to try yoga. All I could think was hippies, and, as much as I respect them, I have never seen a fat hippy. You would think that would urge me to try it, but I figured that it was the lack of processed food and the whole vegan thing that kept them lean.

It wasn't until I actually attended a class that I learned differently. No, you may not be burning a TON of calories, and I don't recommend this alone for a huge amount of weight loss, but make sure you are doing this so the muscles that are building, and yes, any exercise at a large weight is going to build muscles, will be leaner and longer rather than bulky. Bulky muscles mean bigger looking.

I would recommend trying yoga in your home first, and not just sun salutations (those are the ones that are *super simple!*) I recommend waiting on the class just from my own experience. At twenty-six, and about two-hundred-and-seventy-five pounds, I thought, oh so wrongly, that yoga was supposed to be easy.

I walked into a class of about fifteen women who, if they were a day, they were over seventy! Ha Ha! This was going to be a breeze! I have never been *so* wrong! The class started off simple. Breathe in . . . breathe out. Breathe in the positive; breathe out the negative. Can do! Then there was some basic stretching. Reach for your toes (You didn't have to grab them, just aim in their general direction), and breathe.

Reach for the sky and release the negative. Wow! I like this!

Now, put your elbows on the floor, your hands flat against your lower back, raise your shoulders, loosen your neck, raise your shoulders off the floor, lean back, roll your legs up, feet pointing to the sky, contract your stomach muscles . . . and breathe.

Huh? What happened? As I struggled with the final instruction, you know, the whole 'breathing' thing, my face red from lack of oxygen (or the rush of blood) and sweating from exertion, I looked over to see these, 'seasoned' ladies just *flowing* through the movements.

As much as this may be a visual you don't want, these old folks could contort themselves in ways unimaginable! . . . AND STILL BREATHE! So, yeah . . . Start with the yoga where you feel comfortable!

*When you go to the gym, expect pain

No pain, ALL weight gain. Don't push yourself to a heart attack, but don't be a wimp and quit at the first cramp you get when you are jogging. You are going to feel muscle pain. SUCK IT UP! Exercising isn't going to always be fun. There are times that it is going to hurt. You have to learn your limits.

You are going to have trouble breathing. It isn't going to be a walk in the park (okay, well, maybe some days . . .). You are going to get tired. You are going to huff and puff. You are going to get side cramps. A trick to getting rid of a cramp is to breathe out a few times like you are blowing out a ton of candles, while you dig your hand into the side where it hurts. Sounds painful, I know, but some pain is necessary for you success.

Be sure to stretch and walk a bit before exercising. Be sure to stretch and cool-down *after* you exercise. Push yourself. You aren't competing with others, you are competing with yourself. Push yourself a step further each day.

*OUCH!

Warning! The first day after exercise, more than likely, you are going to be SORE! Not just, 'Oh, that was a twinge . . ." kind of sore. I'm talking about, "Holy smack! What the heck did I do to myself???" kind of sore. It is a part of doing what you gotta do.

DO stretch. DO exercise. DO NOT think that if you don't exercise the next day the pain will go away. Not so, my achy friend. It doesn't work that way. If you don't exercise the next day, or stretch, you will be even MORE sore the following day. I can guarantee you, from experience. I know what it feels like to be so sore that when you have to use the restroom, the squat to the toilet KILLS!

I know what it feels like when you wake up that next morning, forgetting that you have kicked your own butt the day before, and try to get out of bed as usual. IT SUCKS . . . but, so does having to shop in the plus-size department.

*Word of Warning . . . also known as WOW

The first two weeks of exercising sucks. No, not just because you aren't used to exerting that amount of energy. Not because you are finding you have muscles in strange places you didn't even know you had, by their soreness. Not because the fact that the whole, "You are going to feel so much more energy!" doesn't happen until about the third week, but for an absolutely HORRIBLE reason that even a seasoned pro like me gets messed up on.

You get the jelly shakes. Your muscles start to appear and it feels like your fat seems to separate from that new muscle, leading to the shake effect. Even worse, clothes may actually seem *tighter!* Unflippin'-believable, I know! To deprive yourself of all your food indulgences and go through the misery of it all, just to FEEL FATTER?!? I kid you not!

I hated that I began building muscle in my arms, but the fat was still there. Waving was so not attractive. My arm would continue waving even after my hand had stopped!

Some people may not go through this, lucky them, but on my journey, my friends and I experienced this.

Melissa Mathis

I had a full bout of this. Unfortunately, I was the largest in my group, so this part of my experience lasted longer than theirs. It was so frustrating to go through, although it was nice to have them going through the same with me at the same time, until, they got through it before I did. So NOT FUN! I was lucky to have the desire to push myself and get through it.

In all honesty though, this was a terrible time. I went through the whole, 'It's not fair!' whine, but thankfully made it through. After about the third week, your body begins to figure it out and starts to change. No matter how hard it is, no matter what, PERSERVERE! DO NOT GIVE UP! I guarantee, you will appreciate it!

*Coffee

Drinking coffee is a GREAT way to increase your energy. We all know that. It has been proven by various studies that drinking coffee before working out leads to the ability to burn more calories. I think we all know this. How many times have we had our coffee and suddenly cleaning the house gets done so much faster than before? Imagine what it is like to drink coffee before working out. Exactly!

*Music

I am *totally* behind when it comes to technology. I was graduating to CD's when the rest of the world was moving on to MP3's. I still remember jogging around the track, well, walking with a bounce, trying to hold my arm steady so the CD wouldn't skip.

The great thing is, now-a-days, even my dad has an MP3 player, and almost any song ever made is available online. When making your collection, make sure to use upbeat songs. I love Patsy Cline, thanks Dad, but trying to work out to "Crazy" is not going to be too effective. Angry songs are also great. I lost the first fifty pounds with the use of anger! A song with a good beat is a great way to motivate you and make the time go faster.

Music is also a great way to test if you are pushing yourself hard enough. If you are able to belt out the tunes as you are on the elliptical machine, you aren't breathing hard enough, which means you aren't pushing yourself hard enough!

There *is* a great use for the slower songs. They are great for stretching . . . remember to stretch!

*Keep rhythm AND TIME

Use a kitchen timer to give yourself a certain amount of time to clean each room. Blast the music and shake your groove thing as you vacuum. Movement is exercise. Cleaning is exercise. Look there! Multi-tasking! Setting the time not only makes you clean faster, you get a better workout and more accomplished in a shorter time.

You know how on television, they have the perfect song for each moment? One of my fantasies is to be rich enough to hire someone who knows every song and would walk around with me and play the perfect song for my day.

But, until that day, I have my MP3 player. I even have a special tutu I wear when I clean. It looks funky, but it makes belting out, 'Girls just wanna have fu-un!' as I clean a lot more exciting.

*H-2-OHHH

Water is SUPER important to weight loss and overall health. Think about it. Approximately two-thirds of our body is water. The coolest thing I read is that your metabolism is majorly boosted when you drink a cup of water with six cubes of ice. Being the extremist I am, well, if one cup of water increases your metabolism for thirty minutes, wouldn't drinking ice water ALL day keep your metabolism revved the whole day? How *easy* is that!

Drink at least two liters of water per day. Sounds easy, I know, but way harder than it seems. Drink at least one bottle of water—16 ounces—before any other drink. Try to drink your water amount early because the later you drink it, the more interrupted sleep you get. The more water you drink, the better.

Drink a cup of water before eating any food. Then, between each bite, take a sip. One, it is conducive to better manners. Two, it will fill your stomach sooner, while still being able to enjoy the food you want to eat. Finally, it is an easier way to fit in your water.

*Vitamins and Minerals

Take a multivitamin each morning. I'm not making your diet for you, but most people don't eat all the nutrients they need, whether or not they are dieting. It will also help with your craving.

P.S. Calcium, B complex and omega 3's are my friends!

Always check with your doctor before taking any supplements.

*Never skip breakfast!

Have you ever heard that we should eat like a king for breakfast, a prince for lunch and a pauper for dinner? Yet, we tend to do it in the exact opposite order, eating the most closest to when we go to bed.

I try to eat 190 calories for this all important meal. This boosts my metabolism in the morning. Not only that, but try to eat the bulk of whatever calories I am going to eat earlier in the day. This allows more time before sleeping to burn the calories off.

*DO NOT EAT BEFORE BED!!!

Duh . . . Let's see, dinner tends to be the biggest meal of our day (which it shouldn't but let's be real), and then we to sleep soon afterwards. Really? And we wonder why we are such a "large" society.

*DO NOT keep eating until you are full!

If you follow the tips of eating slowly, sipping water and eating with your less dominate hand, this should be easier. Stop often as you are eating to check with yourself, "Okay stomach, you still growling?" If the answer is no, STOP EATING. Yes, you will have to eat more often, SMALLER amounts, but, the food is still there, and doesn't it feel great to have just eaten and not feel bloated and nauseous?

*Use your less dominate hand when you eat

Sounds simple, right? Go ahead, try it! Not so easy, is it? You have to concentrate more on what and how you are eating. It will slow you down. Great! More time for your stomach to register that you aren't hungry anymore!

*Use smaller plates and the salad fork or a kid's utensil

In the beginning it is sooooo frustrating, but you will get used to it. Smaller plates fool you into thinking you are eating more than you are. Be real, you have fooled yourself for quite some time now. Now, use that ability to your advantage.

*On the subject of children's utensils

Moms, this is mainly for you. *Do not* eat your kid's leftovers. I know you know what I am talking about. You know, the chicken nugget from their emotional meal, the rest of the roll they didn't finish, the other half of the peanut butter and jelly sandwich they didn't want. It's commendable that you don't want to waste food or the money you spent, but, you also don't want to be a cow. Just because you may not be eating a full serving, doesn't mean the calories don't count! You choose.

When my sister, the one with the amazing children, started her experience, she kept track of how many calories she was eating on her 'normal' days, and found out that she was eating an average of a whopping 470 calories outside of her 'meals' that she didn't realize.

*Experiment

Try new fruits, veggies and recipes. You don't want to get bored with your food. Even if the food is something you love, such as pizza, if you eat it every day, you are going to get sick of it. It is the same with healthy food.

Let's be honest, we are all about being honest in here. More than likely YOU WILL MISS YOUR FOOD. If you are expecting the diet version to taste as good as the original, keep dreaming. Suck it up. Eat diet food, or eat something else.

If having your food tasting great is so important that you would chose to have that New York style pizza over the awesome life you are aiming for, eat it. IT IS YOUR CHOICE THE LIFE YOU LIVE! Your success, your happiness, is in your hands.

*Mirrors

Remember, mirrors are a great tool in losing weight. Whenever possible, eat in front of a mirror.

WARNING:

You may be shocked and mortified. Not only when we are alone do we tend to eat more, we tend to eat *way* more, and, well, slovenly. Watch yourself, catch yourself, fix yourself. Eating with manners means eating slower, taking smaller bites. Not only does it look better, it also allows your stomach to register that there is food in it before you have eaten beyond its limit.

Go back to the exercise where you are supposed to observe people who are where you want to be. As you watch them, no, we are *not* stalking, we are *observing,* notice what they look like when they are eating. Do you see them shoveling food in the mouth? Do you see them with their plate piled high with junk food? Of course not.

Now, look in the mirror as you eat. Do you look like that? Do you look like the person who is already at your goal? Maybe not yet, but emulate the behavior that you want to become a part of your own demeanor. As you look in the mirror, find some positive differences you notice since beginning this experience and smile!

*Choo! Choo!

I'm sure we all have heard how chewing each bite twenty-three times is great for digestion. Now we also know it is great for weight loss. Again, it goes back to taking time eating.

Okay, okay. I'm not going to say to count EVERY time . . . makes it hard for dinner conversation, but estimate. Over all ENJOY each and every bite you eat. Pay attention to the food that is in your mouth. Enjoy the taste, smell and texture. As with everything in life, take your time and savor the flavor.

*Eat what you want

Sounds crazy, huh? When I first started my experience, I had one cheat day a week. The first week, as I would crave something, I would write it down. I didn't want to miss *anything* on my cheat day.

The first Saturday, the day I had chosen to cheat, I ate worse than I did on day three! I spent the whole day eating, pigging out, going back and forth to the refrigerator. I actually gained three pounds when I weighed myself the following day. What I hated most about myself that day was the fact that I ate things I had craved in the week and put on my list, but by the time Saturday came, I wasn't really craving them anymore; yet, I still ate it all. It was getting a slap in the face from the old me and negating all my hard work during the week.

The next week, I changed it to just a cheat meal. That was a bit better, but it still had that effect that 'the last meal' had when I first started. Then I finally figured it out. I allowed myself two things on my cheat day that I wanted. I allowed myself to eat at birthday parties. I just made sure I had my lovely girdle on when I was there.

In telling yourself that you can never again have a candy bar or ice cream or cheesecake it is like putting a toy on the table in front of a kid and saying, 'Don't touch it. Don't think about it. Don't want it.' What is going to happen? All that kid is going to be able to think about is that toy and want it, and the moment the adult is out of site, that child is going to grab that toy.

Allow yourself some leeway. As always, you are human. Neglect what you want too long, and you will binge. I'm not saying eat *everything* you want, but think in portions and NOT EVERY DAY. I have never eaten one-third of a king size candy bar. Maybe THREE king size candy bars, but NEVER a third. So, when I read, on the package of one of my all-time favorite candy bars, man's gift to women, that one-third is a serving size, well, COME ON NOW! Really??? But, as sad as I am to say this, we have to learn portion control. Read the label and follow directions.

*Your new best friend

You are going to have days. I mean *DAYS.* You know what I am talking about. The days when your stress level seems to be beyond bearable. If you aren't able to keep from the angry munching, don't add to your stress level by trying to not eat anything other than fruits and veggies. This is a *life* change, and if you aren't able to find a way to deal with your stress, if you don't find a way to deal with your stress *while dieting*, you are going to binge and give up. Let's fix this.

If you are frustrated and you aren't finding the strength within yourself to not eat, okay. Popcorn is your *best* friend. Air-popped, plain popcorn is your best choice but, personally, I hate the plain taste. Pop Weaver Kettle corn not only has just about seventy calories per bag, popped, but it has that sweet and salty flavor at the same time! The best thing about it is that it also has enough crunch for the aggravation. Pop and eat . . . then walk.

We are not trying to change your nature, we are tweaking it. Stress is a part of life, a BIG part of life. We have to learn to deal with it in a way that isn't going to mess up your life more than it already is!

There are other alternatives for dealing with stress that helps get that aggression out.

I know it may surprise you, but I come from a long line of 'blunt' people. But, I also come from a long line of 'respect your elders' people. When I was thirteen-years-old, relatives from my 'blunt' side came to visit for a while. My mother warned me that if they said anything that upset me, I couldn't say anything back. Not easy for a teenager. But, she gave me a great tool in losing weight.

At this time, we lived on a ranch with a running track. My mother told me that if I wanted to say something back to them, to excuse myself and go walk the track. In the three weeks they visited, I lost thirteen pounds!

It was one of the first tricks to losing weight that I learned. A punching bag is also great. Just be sure to wear gloves!

*Graffiti yourself beautiful

Dry erase markers are AMAZING! They are great for the motivational reminders of how great you are that you can write on your bathroom mirror. The bathroom mirror is a great place to write something great about yourself each night before you go to bed. Change it often so you don't get used to seeing the same words over and over so you don't even really see them anymore.

Remember, beauty is NOT in the eye of the beholder, it is in the eyes of the beheld. Simply put, see the beauty in yourself. If you feel the world is against you, why should you join that team? That's a guaranteed loss, and I don't mean weight loss!

I don't want to hear that crap of, "Oh, there's nothing about me that is beautiful." Really? Shut up, sit down (in front of the mirror), and look. I guarantee you there is something wonderful about yourself. Find it. Then, use that awesome dry-erase marker and write it down.

Another great use for the amazing markers is reminders. I don't know about you, but my will power is weakest at night. I will literally be lying in bed thinking about what food I have in my fridge. During the day I am able to keep myself busy, to keep my mind occupied; but, the night, oh the night is my weakness. Remember, calories eaten in the dark still count!

To remind myself, I leave the light over the stove on and have attached a dry erase board to my refrigerator and cupboard to tell me to *go to bed* and to remind myself of what I REALLY want.

As much as I hate to admit it, I will often put the name of someone I am super competitive with or just, well, really not liking at that time on the board. Yes, we are supposed to let go of things that anger us, but if you do have it, use it properly. Anger or frustration, focused in the proper direction can lead to positive results for you! Use your handy-dandy-dry-erase marker to remind you!

*Commercials are not our friends!

Recording our shows so we can fast-forward through commercials is awesome! Have you ever done good all day on your healthy eating and then you come home, watch television, and then, suddenly, you can't get pizza out of your mind? Hmmmm . . . I wonder where that idea came from. In our new home, I have yet to figure out how to record my shows.

Right now, as I type, I have the television on for background noise. There is now a restaurant that is having some chocolate lava flow. I was doing great today, yet suddenly I have this insane craving for chocolate! The only blessing I have is the fact that it is too late to run to the store to go buy chocolate! It is amazing how susceptible our minds are to suggestion, yet it seems to be the bad suggestions that seem to stick with us the most. I don't see a commercial of someone working out at the gym and get a sudden hankering to hop onto a stationary bike!

Record the shows you like to watch. Skip through the commercials. Hey! What's that? Wow! MORE time found in your day. Congratulations! Use it wisely!

*Rewards

Okay, so a gold star sticker worked when you were a kid, why not now? One thing teachers are right on track with is marking success on a chart. Marking good days on a calendar where you can see your continuous success. When you hit a certain amount of days, reward yourself. A few weeks, celebrate!

Here is the clincher though. When you have reached a goal, reward yourself with something *other than food*! Isn't it amazing how we have made food our reward? It's sad that we have to stop and think hard about what could be a reward, once you tell yourself it can't be food.

Maybe there is a movie out that you have been wanting to see. Maybe there is a new coffee shop. Maybe there is a book (ahem) out that you want. Maybe your reward could be a sexy pair of panties. Well, for you men reading this, it could be something different, like a power tie, a new gym bag . . . or not. Whatever floats your boat and motivates you.

*Tangible weight-loss recording

Seeing the number on the scale go down is great, even if it is just a small amount, but, when you have been pushing yourself hard and denying yourself your comfort foods just to see that you have *only* lost five to ten pounds is frustrating. A number is just a number, until you show yourself exactly what that number symbolizes.

For every five pounds you lose, go to the store and get a five-pound weight disc. Put it in a back pack. Five pounds, especially when you have thirty times that to lose, doesn't *sound* like much, but when you put it in the bag and wear it, you *feel* it. When you get up to ten or fifteen pounds in the bag, you REALLY feel it.

This is a better way than just seeing numbers on a scale to keep motivated. It is also a great way to keep you on the right path. When you are tempted to eat something that will COMPLETELY blow your work to smithereens, put on the backpack and walk around for ten minutes. After you take it off, walk around for one more minute. Notice the difference? NOW make your decision.

*The 'I ams'

I have read and heard that the following plan works. It is VERY easy to do, and if there is a chance that it works, why not try it? In the short time that I have done the plan, it seems to have worked for me. I got a digital voice recorder and listed what I *really* want. The worst part of this plan is recording it. For an hour and twenty-five minutes I repeated the same lines over and over. This is a great time to use the list of what it *really* is that you want from yourself, what you want in your life. Include what you want physically, as well as mentally, emotionally and materialistically. I walked around my block over and over pretending I was on a cell phone repeating, "I am thin, I am beautiful, I am intelligent, I am calm, I am energetic . . ." and so on. Then, as I am about to fall asleep, I put on the headphones and listen to it until it shuts itself off at the end. Anything this easy to motivate us, why not try?

Note to you: Be careful what you wish for, and make sure to keep your words positive!

*Sleep

I have a habit of buying rechargeable batteries. They are a great idea, especially when I follow the last idea and use my recorder each night. The problem is, I almost always forget to charge them so they will be ready when the one I am using needs to be charged. I end up having to go buy more batteries, not great for the environment or the wallet. Our bodies are similar to these rechargeable batteries. If you don't recharge it, you don't get enough sleep, it's not going to work. The problem with our body though, we can't run to the store to grab another one.

Get seven to nine hours of sleep. Your body needs it. Period. If you have a habit of only five to six hours a night of sleep, don't try to hop to nine hours. Add ten minutes every couple of days to go to bed earlier. No action films before bed! Dim your lighting half an hour before heading to bed. Turn the alarm clock away from you. A battery can't run without charge, and neither can you!

* Newsflash

YOU ARE HUMAN!

Humans aren't perfect. You are going to make mistakes, have slip ups, become overwhelmed. I'm here to tell you, that it's OKAY. What isn't okay is having a slip up, feeling like a failure, then quitting. In fact, let's use that slip up. RECORD IT IN YOUR JOURNAL. Just because you don't write it down doesn't mean it didn't happen.

Ashamed? Great! Guilty? Wonderful! Write down how you feel. Now, was whatever you ate in the five minutes it took to eat it worth how you feel? Of course not. YOU HAVE NOT FAILED! Great news! You have just added more ammunition to your arsenal to fight the battle of the bulge.

Any time you are tempted, turn to this page in your journal; read it, feel it, remember it. THEN make your decision.

*Let it go

Stress is gonna happen. As a human being there are a few things we can totally plan on; breathing, eating, and stress. Some stresses, we have NO control over. But, we do have control over how we respond, not *react*, but *respond* to it.

Allowing ourselves to sit and worry isn't going to change it. Do what you can, and what you have no control over, give it to whatever higher power you believe in. Then, get busy. An idle hand is a stressing mind. A stressed out mind is a fat body.

We are absolutely amazing at making excuses for ourselves, so let's try this for others. Someone cuts you off driving. Okay, that sucks. But, think of how stupid you look from the outside yelling to a person who cannot hear you and more than likely can't see you. Let's change that.

Instead of thinking that the person who cut you off is a jerk who doesn't care about or respect others, maybe it is a man or woman whose spouse is at home with their sick child who is throwing up all over the place and they are rushing home with the medicine. Wow! A hero! Cheer him on. Wish him luck!

Are you a in a rush at the supermarket and you get into the express lane but all it does is make you want to 'express' your frustration when they have put a trainee as the cashier and they are slower than a turtle in molasses? Man, that sucks. Getting mad and making negative comments is going to remedy the situation, right? Getting frustrated is going to make the cashier work faster . . . ? Exactly.

Imagine you are that new trainee. The poor kid is probably terrified of messing up and doing the best he can. If you say something negative, is that going to make him go faster? He'd probably react like most people, including you, react to stress; he would just mess up more. Instead, how about you ease his stress, give him a smile, or just breathe.

Now, don't YOU feel better? If you stressing isn't going to change the results, find a way to let it go . . . DON'T HEAD STRAIGHT FOR THE FRIDGE TO EAT! Look at your list of "What to do instead of aimlessly eating." Okay . . . now proceed.

*So, Lyssa, what's the diet?

Okay, okay. I know what you're thinking. "Man, I'm almost at the end of this book on how to lose weight and I have yet to see a diet . . . hmmm . . . kinda strange." Well, please put your finger on this page as a placeholder and look at the cover of this book . . . don't worry, I'll be here when you get back . . .

Welcome back. Okay. Did you look? Did you see it? That is your answer. As the title tells you, "It Ain't No Darn Diet." Now, let's look at the basics of what most people know already. If you remember from math class in school, when the teachers are telling you about how to use calculators, it is all about "G.I.G.O" or, Garbage in, Garbage Out. We all know the way to lose weight is less calories consumed than calories used. Eat bad, well, the result will be bad. Eat good, then good results. Diet is a *huge* percentage of weight loss. I understand the question I get of, "What diet did you do?" but it is not a simple answer. There wasn't just one diet. Like I said, you name the diet, and I have tried it. *And*, almost every diet works . . . for a while. But then your body gets used to it and it works less. So you change it up. And the new one will work. And then it doesn't so, guess what, you change it again. There are a lot of great diets out there. The super low carb ones are highly effective, but to maintain for too long and keep your friends? Well, you will have no friends left (lack of too many carbs makes you REALLY cranky).

The shake one is great because you know what exactly to eat (bad for the noses of the families of those affected by lactose, and I like chewing!). The soup one is also highly effective, but for long term, well, after about a week and a half, you won't be able to swallow the soup, even though you are hungry.

Cyclical calories is one of my favorites because you make a list of how many calories you can have each day, ranging from seven hundred to seventeen hundred making sure that it is a different amount each day. My rule of thumb: I never do less than twelve hundred calories per day for more than three days in a row. This makes my body go into famine mode and hold on to EVERY calorie you eat! Regardless of the day, if I wanted to eat a candy bar, I could, I just had to count those calories against the amount I had left. This diet, mixed with the basic food pyramid we learned in first grade, is actually one of my favorites.

My brother does the "bag diet" which incorporates the cyclical calories with making all the food with the right amount of calories the night before and putting it all into a bag. You can eat all the food in that bag the next day, all at once, over time, at the end, at the beginning, but, no more than what is in the bag. This is actually a cool one because you don't have to think the whole day about what you are going to eat, or how many calories are in what you are eating.

Overall, there are so many diets out there to try. I try each one for a while and see what works for me. I give each about two weeks to see the results. If they are good and I want to continue on it, do. If they aren't what I want, I switch it up. I can always come back to a diet that works well in the beginning and then slows down later. I shock my body. I don't let it know what to expect. I pick and choose. I don't get bored. I make it in two week increments so I know there is a beginning and end. This *is* a lifestyle change, but dieting on the same diet forever isn't fun. I may love pizza, but if i had pizza every day, I would get sick of it. Same with this.

The most important thing to understand is, like I said before, your fat isn't the problem, it is a symptom. Losing weight is more about psychology than physiology. Emotions muck us up. Stress makes us fat, well, our reaction to stress makes us fat. Pay attention to what you are reading, and what your body is telling you and you will succeed!

*Don't want to be *that* again!

One thing that people who have perpetually dieted have a huge problem with, myself included, is keeping weight lost, off. We are so intent on losing the weight that we forget that there is going to come a time where we only need to maintain. Sounds simple, huh? Once you get to your goal, YOU ARE NOT DONE. It does not mean that you can just forget doing all you were doing to get to where you are. It means that you have to train yourself to eat healthy.

If all these tips are followed, portion control should be a habit. You should be able to eye-ball what a REAL serving size is and estimate your calories without having to write everything down. Just remember, the stomach expands, and the more often you expand it more than necessary, the more you are going to eat larger amounts on a regular basis.

I'll say it again, WEIGH YOURSELF *EVERY* DAY. This is of utmost importance. Speaking from experience, unfortunately, I have lost a MASSIVE AMOUNT of weight and promised myself I would never be fat again to wake up one day and realize that I was fat . . . again.

Of course . . . The warning signs were there; you know, the shorter skirts disappearing into the back of the closet; Non-stretch jeans joining them shortly after. In fact, most non-stretch clothes joined them.

One major key to keeping the weight off is weighing yourself every day. It is WAY easier to lose one to two pounds than it is ten to twenty. When you see you have gained weight, do what is necessary to get it back off immediately!

*My journey continues

I'm not yet to my goal. I am still going through my experience. I have about thirty more pounds to go, and as much as that may seem, compared to how much I have lost, I know I can do it. This is the HARDEST time. Not only am I fighting my body, fighting the final THIRTY, my life has way beyond the usual amount of stress.

My usual M.O. for stress is to sleep and eat. I cannot do that. That is *not* going to get me to where I need to be. FOOD IS NOT THE ANSWER! So, I am fighting, tooth and nail, against my instincts to revert to my natural comforts of food and sleep.

It isn't that I *won't* fail. It is that I CANNOT fail. That is my choice. This is my life. I have to choose what is best for me. Don't think I am just talking the talk. I am here with you, walking the walk each step, feeling the pain, accepting my blame of my place in life and knowing that I will be able to accept the kudos for my success.

Come, join me.

Tips:

* Make plans for the future. Start now!
* Make a list of things that sucked and what you have kept yourself from
* Make a list of reasons to stay fat
* Two days of your 'normal' eating and exercise, recorded
* 1 ½ hours of gorging
* Write how you feel after the binge
* Write how you will feel when you succeed
* First weigh-in should be in the morning
* Weigh yourself at the same time in the same clothes each day
* Beware of the PMS bloat!
* Create short term goals as well
* Take pictures from all angles
* Make a list of what you can do instead of aimlessly eating
* Make 'To Do' lists
* Get the your least-liked tasks done first
* List *exactly* what you want in your life physically, mentally, and materialistically
* Wear tight clothes
* Tell people who you are around often that you are trying to lose weight
* Clip and *read* motivational stories
* Be your own cheerleader

* Clean, Clean, Clean!
* Get organized
* Get a friend to try these new experiences with you
* Put yourself around positive people
* Dress well
* Not so much boobage!

Tips Continued:

* Get comfortable gym clothes
* Get rid of clothes when they become too big for you
* Keep one pair of non-stretch pants from your biggest size
* Make a list of people you admire and why
* Practice *now* who you want to become
* Put yourself first
* Be happy already. Appreciate *all* successes
* Smile
* Fake it 'til you make it
* Appreciate a compliment and respond correctly
* Aim for 'Slut'
* Make time for exercise
* Play with your kids (or someone else's)
* Keep your gym bag in the car
* Park further away from your destination
* Exercise is great, *any* exercise
* Chose a gym wisely
* Find your ambition
* Pick the exercises that are right for you
* Try different classes and exercises

* Maximize your workouts by changing the exercise you are doing every 15 minutes
* Wear a pedometer
* Yoga/Stretching . . . Brilliant!
* When you go to the gym, expect some pain and discomfort
* Expect soreness after working out. Be sure to work out the next day, regardless of how sore you are.
* Be prepared for the 'jelly-shakes'. It will go away usually by week three
* Drink coffee before working out

Tips Continued:

* Listen to upbeat music as you work out
* Use a kitchen timer and time yourself cleaning
* Drink at least two liters of water each day
* Vitamins are your friends
* Never skip breakfast. Eat at least 190 calories for this meal
* Do not eat right before bed
* Do not keep eating until you are full
* Use your less dominate hand when you eat
* Use smaller plates and the salad fork or kids' utensil when eating
* Do not eat your children's left-over food
* Try new foods you have never had before
* Whenever possible, eat while looking into a mirror
* Chew your food twenty-three times per bite
* Eat what you want—in proper portion size

* Popcorn (check the label) is great for the times you want to aggression-eat
* Use a dry-erase marker to write inspirations on your bathroom mirror
* Record the shows you want to watch and fast forward through commercials
* Reward yourself with something other than food when you have achieved a goal
* Buy a 5lb weight and put in a back pack for each 5 pounds lost
* Write what you want to be in the form of 'I am . . ."
* Get 8-9 hours of sleep
* Don't quit if you slip up once
* Deal with your stress
* Choose a diet, and switch it up
* When you reach your goal, still weigh each day to maintain
* Join me and let's succeed together!

Plus Size Panty Problems

The pooje, the second roll, the overhang small children could shade themselves with in the summer-yes, I am talking about the lovely, lower stomach. I'm not as concerned with the lower stomach in itself, but in the way in which we adorn it. There are two typical schools of thought on how a "voluptuous" woman should go about choosing the panty style for them.

The word "panty" is really quite deceiving. "Panty" makes the article of clothing seem so dainty. Say it with a British accent, and it seems like some type of sugary pastry. When it comes to the panties in my size, 'dainty' would be the last word I would associate with them. *Gargantuous, humungous, parachute;* these are the words that come to my mind!

I currently have a wide assortment of the lovely, world-famous, 'granny panties' in varying shades of white. Every so often the creators of these monstrosities remember that they are being made for women and they'll feminine 'em up with a ton of itty-bitty flowers. As previously mentioned, the bigger the dress, the bigger the flower, both those in the panty industry take the opposite approach.

They produce undergarments with flowers so small they begin to appear as polk-a-dots lost in the vast expanse of my rear, a natural source of jiggling that, if walking in just undergarments alone, could blind innocent bystanders!

Not only are these panties dull in color, there is no real style to them. It seems the maker's theory is 'tuck and cover,' meaning: suck in and cover as much as possible. In theory, the 'suck-in' panties are a great idea, but you have to wonder, what happens to the surplus fat for which there just isn't enough room? You are right; the 'underpants overhang.' You know, that lovely bulge of fat that isn't as present when you are not wearing the suck-in panties. Some makers have tried to curb this problem by lengthening our underpants, seeming to use enough material to clothe a small family. This extra material creates the 'under-the-boob' effect which makes any woman feel, oh so sexy.

Then we have the polar opposite school of thought. This is the idea that we, and again, by 'we' I mean voluptuous women, deserve to wear the same style of panties as those quite smaller than us. I agree, although I am thankful that I cannot see myself from behind. There are reasons I'd never get one of those three-way mirrors. There are just some sides of myself to which I would rather remain oblivious.

My favorites are the super lacy, not too high on the top, but above the end of your butt cheeks, panties.

Now these *really* make a girl feel like a woman. The only downfall to this style is the fact that quite a large amount of material is seemingly permanently wedged into the 'abyss'. But, if you aren't doing a whole lot of walking, they are wonderful. They also cover the wonderful back fat, or as I call it, my second stomach. The way I discovered mine was quite by accident.

My sister had one of those three-way mirrors of horror, and I had bought my first pair of thongs. I made the mistake of trying them on and actually looking into that mirror. To this day, I am not sure what possessed me to look, but that was the day I had to admit I was a pretty big girl; not a pretty girl, a *pretty BIG girl!* I had lost the thong. I looked and looked, but all I could find was a purple string around my waist. Going to pull of the purple thread, I found, or rather, I felt, where my thong had wandered. And yet, I still looked, inspected the image in the mirror and discovered that I didn't look *anything* like the models on my underwear package. The models had a dip before their behinds began, mine wasn't, well, it just wasn't as *defined.* In fact, there wasn't much definition to where my back ended and my butt began. I came to the conclusion that thongs just weren't meant for me.

Then I decided I'd try the silk, non-stretch kind that had the stretchy string at the sides, which ended up creating a double roll effect on each side of the string. Not as sexy and flattering as I had expected. If that didn't happen, I would have had the problem as I did when I wore 'low-riders'.

I understand now that low-riders have their name for a reason. Unfortunately for me, they became 'lower riders,' rolling down to the bottom of my belly, providing no support, completely unlike the support I'd gotten used to with my granny panties.

I'm waiting for the day that panty professionals create a panty that can lift, tuck, suck and shape all in a sexy design!